Air Fryer Toaster Oven Recipes For Daily Healthy Meals

Quick And Affordable Recipes To Boost Your Air Fryer Toaster Oven Diet And Stay Fit

Eva Morris

TABLE OF CONTENT

Cinnamon Cream Doughnuts.. 7

Sausage Frittata... 9

Potato Jalapeno Hash... 11

Bread Rolls...13

Cheddar & Cream Omelet.. 15

Zucchini Omelet... 17

Eggs In Avocado Cups... 19

Cinnamon French Toasts.. 21

Savory French Toast...23

Cheddar Mustard Toasts..26

Ricotta Toasts With Salmon.. 28

Zucchini Fritters.. 30

Air Fryer Hard-Boiled Eggs.. 32

Easy Air Fryer Baked Eggs With Cheese............................ 34

Bacon-And-Eggs Avocado.. 36

Double-Dipped Mini Cinnamon Biscuits............................38

Foolproof Air Fryer Bacon... 42

Merit Age Eggs.. 44

Easy Air Fryer Buttermilk Biscuits.................................. 46

Breakfast Pizza... 49

Easy Bacon...51

Chicken And Asparagus...52

Spinach And Olives...54

- ½ cup tomato puree... 54

- 2cups black olives pitted and halved............................. 54

- 3celery stalks; chopped... 54

- 1red bell pepper; chopped...54

- Two tomatoes; chopped..54

- Salt and black pepper..54

Broccoli Stew... 56

Turkey And Bok Choy... 57

Breakfast Potatoes.. 59

Breakfast Egg Rolls.. 61

Air Fryer Sausage Breakfast Casserole..............................64

Air Fryer Egg In Hole.. 66

Air Fryer Baked Egg Cups With Spinach & Cheese...................67

Breakfast Casserole..69

Cheesy Bacon And Egg Hash..71

Bacon Cheddar Biscuits.. 73

Potato Hash Brown Casserole... 76

Sweet Potato Casserole..79

Cheesy Garlic Sweet Potatoes... 81

Blueberry Muffins.. 83

Eggs, Bacon, Tomato, And Cheese Bake............................... 85

Bacon Bombs... 88

Morning Potatoes.. 90

Breakfast Pockets...*92*

Avocado Flautas...*94*

Cheese Sandwiches...*96*

Sausage Cheese Wraps..*98*

Chicken Omelet...*100*

Sausage Burritos..*102*

Sausage Patties..*104*

Spicy Sweet Potato Hash...*106*

this book has been derived from various sources. Please consult a licensed professional before attempting any techniques outlined in this book.

By reading this document, the reader agrees that under no circumstances is the author responsible for any losses, direct or indirect, which are incurred as a result of the use of information contained within this document, including, but not limited to, — errors, omissions, or inaccuracies.

Cinnamon Cream Doughnuts

Preparation Time: 10 minutes

Cooking Time: 8 minutes

Serving: 4

Ingredients:

- 1/2 cup Sugar
- 2 1/2 tbsp. butter
- Two large egg yolks
- 2 1/4 cups all-purpose flour
- 1 1/2 tsp. baking powder
- 1 tsp. salt
- 1/2 cup sour cream
- To garnish
- 1/3 cup white Sugar
- 1 tsp. cinnamon
- 2 tbsp. butter, melted

Directions:

1. Beat egg with sugar and butter in a mixer until creamy, then whisk in flour, salt, baking powder, and sour cream.

2. Mix well until smooth, and then refrigerate the dough for 1 hour. Spread this dough into ½ inch thick circle, and then cut nine large circles out of it.

3. Make the hole at the center of each circle. Place the doughnuts in the Air Fryer basket. Set the Air Fryer basket inside the Air Fryer toaster oven and close the lid. Select the Air Fry mode at 350 degrees F temperature for 8 minutes.

4. Cook the doughnuts in two batches to avoid overcrowding. Mix sugar, cinnamon, and butter and glaze the doughnuts with this mixture. Serve.

Nutrition:

Calories: 387   Protein: 10.6gCarbs: 26.4gFat: 13g

Sausage Frittata

Preparation Time: 10 minutes

Cooking Time: 15 minutes

Serving: 4

Ingredients:

- 1/4-pound sausage, cooked and crumbled
- Four eggs, beaten
- 1/2 cup shredded Cheddar cheese blend
- 2 tbsp. red bell pepper, diced
- One green onion, chopped
- One pinch of cayenne pepper
- cooking spray

Directions:

1. Beat eggs with cheese, sausage, cayenne, onion, and bell pepper in a bowl. Spread the egg mixture in a 6x2 inch baking tray, greased with cooking spray.

2. Set the baking tray inside the Air Fryer toaster oven and close the lid.

3. Select the Bake mode at 360 degrees F temperature for 20 minutes. Slice and serve.

Nutrition:

Calories: 212   Protein: 17.3 garbs: 14.6gFat: 11.8g

Potato Jalapeno Hash

Preparation Time: 15 minutes

Cooking Time: 24 minutes

Serving: 4

Ingredients:

- 1 1/2 lbs. potatoes, peeled and diced
- 1 tbsp. olive oil
- One red bell pepper, seeded and diced
- One small onion, chopped
- One jalapeno, seeded and diced
- 1/2 tsp. olive oil
- 1/2 tsp. taco seasoning mix
- 1/2 tsp. ground cumin
- salt and black pepper to taste

Directions:

1. Soak the potato in cold water for 20 minutes, and then drain them. Toss the potatoes with 1 tbsp.—olive oil. Spread them in the Air Fryer basket. Set the Air Fryer basket inside the Air Fryer toaster

oven and close the lid.

2. Select the Air Fry mode at 370 degrees F temperature for 18 minutes. And meanwhile, toss onion, pepper, olive oil, taco seasoning, and all other ingredients in a salad bowl.

3. Add this vegetable mixture to the Air Fryer basket, and it returns it to the oven. Continue cooking at 356 degrees F for 6 minutes. Serve warm.

Nutrition:

Calories: 242   Protein: 8.9gCarbs: 36.8gFat: 14.4g

Bread Rolls

Preparation Time: 10 minutes

Cooking Time: 39 minutes

Serving: 8

Ingredients:

- 8 Bread Slices
- 2 Potatoes boiled and mashed
- 1 tsp. Ginger grated
- 1 tbsp. Coriander powder
- 1 tsp. Cumin powder
- 1/2 tsp. Chili powder
- 1/2 tsp. Garam Masala
- 1/2 tsp. Dry Mango powder
- 1&1/2 tsp. Salt
- 1 Large Bowl of Water
- Cooking Oil

Directions:

1. Mix mashed potatoes with ginger and all the spices. Divide this mixture into 16 balls and keep them aside. Slice the bread

slices into half to get 16 rectangles.

2. Dip each in water for 1 second, then place one potato ball at the center and wrap the slice around it. Place half of these wrapped balls in the Air Fryer basket and spray them with cooking oil.

3. Set the Air Fryer basket inside the Air Fryer toaster oven and close the lid. Select the Air Fry mode at 390 degrees F temperature for 18 minutes. Flip the balls after 10 minutes of cooking, and then continue cooking.

4. Cook the remaining balls in the same manner. Serve fresh.

Nutrition:

Calories: 331   Protein: 14.8gCarbs: 46gFat: 2.5g

Cheddar & Cream Omelet

Preparation Time: 10 minutes

Cooking Time: 8 minutes

Serving: 2

Ingredients:

- Four eggs
- 1/4 cup cream
- Salt and ground black pepper
- 1/4 cup Cheddar cheese, grated

Directions:

1. In a bowl, add the eggs, cream, salt, and black pepper and beat well.
2. Place the egg mixture into a small baking pan.
3. Press the Power Button of Air Fry Oven and turn the dial to select the Air Fry mode.
4. Press the Time button and again turn the dial to set the cooking time to 8 minutes.

5. Now push the Temp button and rotate the dial to set the temperature at 350 degrees F.

6. Press the Start/Pause button to start.

7. When the unit beeps to show that it is preheated, open the lid.

8. Arrange the pan over the Wire Rack and insert it in the oven.

9. After 4 minutes, sprinkle the omelet with cheese evenly.

10. Cut the omelet into two portions and serve hot.

11. Cut into equal-sized wedges and serve hot.

Nutrition:

Calories 202, Fat 15.1 g, Carbs 1.8 g,

Protein 14.8 g

Zucchini Omelet

Preparation Time: 15 minutes

Cooking Time: 14 minutes

Serving: 2

Ingredients:

- One teaspoon butter
- One zucchini, julienned
- Four eggs
- 1/4 teaspoon fresh basil, chopped
- 1/4 teaspoon red pepper flakes, crushed
- Salt and ground black pepper

Directions:

1. In a skillet, melt the butter over medium heat and cook the zucchini for about 3-4 minutes.
2. Remove from the heat and set aside to cool slightly.
3. Meanwhile, in a bowl, mix the eggs, basil, red pepper flakes, salt, and black pepper.

4. Add the cooked zucchini and gently stir to combine.

5. Place the zucchini mixture into a small baking pan.

6. Press the Power Button of Air Fry Oven and turn the dial to select the Air Fry mode.

7. Press the Time button and again turn the dial to set the cooking time to 10 minutes.

8. Now push the Temp button and rotate the dial to set the temperature at 355 degrees F.

9. Press the Start/Pause button to start.

10. When the unit beeps to show that it is preheated, open the lid.

11. Arrange the pan over the Wire Rack and insert it in the oven.

12. Cut the omelet into two portions and serve hot.

Nutrition:

Calories 159, Fat 10.9 g, Carbs 4.1 g, Protein 12.3 g

Eggs In Avocado Cups

Preparation Time: 10 minutes

Cooking Time: 10 minutes

Serving: 2

Ingredients:

- One avocado halved and pitted

- Two large eggs

- Salt and ground black pepper

- Two cooked bacon slices, crumbled

Directions:

1. Carefully scoop out about two teaspoons of flesh from each avocado half.

2. Crack one egg in each avocado half and sprinkle with salt and black pepper.

3. Press the Power Button of Air Fry Oven and turn the dial to select the Air Roast mode.

4. Press the Time button and again turn the dial to set the cooking time to 10 minutes.

5. Now push the Temp button and rotate the dial to set the temperature at 375 degrees F.

6. Press the Start/Pause button to start.

7. When the unit beeps to show that it is preheated, open the lid and line the Sheet Pan with a light grease piece of foil.

8. Arrange avocado halves into the Sheet Pan and insert them in the oven.

9. Top each avocado half with bacon pieces and serve.

Nutrition:

Calories 300, Fat 26.6 g, Carbs 9 g, Protein 9.7 g

Cinnamon French Toasts

Preparation Time: 10 minutes

Cooking Time: 5 minutes

Serving: 2

Ingredients:

- Two eggs
- 1/4 cup whole milk
- Three tablespoons sugar
- Two teaspoons olive oil
- 1/8 teaspoon vanilla extract
- 1/8 teaspoon ground cinnamon
- Four bread slices

Directions:

1. In a large bowl, mix all the ingredients except bread slices.
2. Coat the bread slices with egg mixture evenly.
3. Press the Power Button of Air Fry Oven and turn the dial to select the Air Fry mode.

4. Press the Time button and again turn the dial to set the cooking time to 6 minutes.

5. Now push the Temp button and rotate the dial to set the temperature at 390 degrees F.

6. Press the Start/Pause button to start.

7. When the unit beeps to show that it is preheated, open the lid and lightly grease the sheet pan.

8. Arrange the bread slices into Air Fry Basket and insert them in the oven.

9. Flip the bread slices once halfway through.

10. Serve warm.

Nutrition:

Calories 238, Fat 10.6 g, Carbs 20.8 g Protein 7.9 g

Savory French Toast

Preparation Time: 10 minutes

Cooking Time: 5 minutes

Serving:

Ingredients:

- 1/4 cup chickpea flour
- Three tablespoons onion, finely chopped
- Two teaspoons green chili, seeded and finely chopped
- 1/2 teaspoon red chili powder
- 1/4 teaspoon ground turmeric
- 1/4 teaspoon ground cumin
- Salt, to taste
- Water
- Four bread slices

Directions:

1. Add all the ingredients except bread slices in a large bowl and mix until a thick mixture form.

2. With a spoon, spread the mixture over both sides of each bread slice.

3. Arrange the bread slices into the lightly greased sheet pan.

4. Press the Power Button of Air Fry Oven and turn the dial to select the Air Fry mode.

5. Press the Time button and again turn the dial to set the cooking time to 5 minutes.

6. Now push the Temp button and rotate the dial to set the temperature at 390 degrees F.

7. Press the Start/Pause button to start.

8. When the unit beeps to show that it is preheated, open the lid and lightly grease the sheet pan.

9. Arrange the bread slices into Air Fry Basket and insert them in the oven.

10. Flip the bread slices once halfway through.

11. Serve warm.

Nutrition:

Calories 151, Fat 2.3 g, Carbs 26.7 g, Protein 6.5 g

Cheddar Mustard Toasts

Preparation Time: 10 minutes

Cooking Time: 10 minutes

Serving: 2

Ingredients:

- Four bread slices
- Two tablespoons cheddar cheese, shredded
- Two eggs, whites, and yolks separated
- One tablespoon mustard
- One tablespoon paprika

Directions:

1. In a clean glass bowl, add the egg whites and beat until they form soft peaks.
2. In another bowl, mix the cheese, egg yolks, mustard, and paprika.
3. Gently fold in the egg whites.
4. Spread the mustard mixture over the toasted bread slices.

5. Press the Power Button of Air Fry Oven and turn the dial to select the Air Fry mode.

6. Press the Time button and again turn the dial to set the cooking time to 10 minutes.

7. Now push the Temp button and rotate the dial to set the temperature at 355 degrees F.

8. Press the Start/Pause button to start.

9. When the unit beeps to show that it is preheated, open the lid and lightly grease the sheet pan.

10. Arrange the bread slices into Air Fry Basket and insert them in the oven.

11. Serve warm.

Nutrition:

Calories 175, Fat 9.4 g, Carbs 13.4 g, Protein 10.6 g

Ricotta Toasts With Salmon

Preparation Time: 10 minutes

Cooking Time: 4 minutes

Serving: 2

Ingredients:

- Four bread slices

- One garlic clove, minced

- 8 oz. ricotta cheese

- One teaspoon lemon zest

- Freshly ground black pepper

- 4 oz. smoked salmon

Directions:

1. In a food processor, add the garlic, ricotta, lemon zest, and black pepper and pulse until smooth.

2. Spread ricotta mixture over the bread slices evenly.

3. Press the Power Button of Air Fry Oven and turn the dial to select the Air Fry mode.

4. Press the Time button and again turn the dial to set the cooking time to 4 minutes.

5. Now push the Temp button and rotate the dial to set the temperature at 355 degrees F.

6. Press the Start/Pause button to start.

7. When the unit beeps to show that it is preheated, open the lid and lightly grease the sheet pan.

8. Arrange the bread slices into Air Fry Basket and insert them in the oven.

9. Top with salmon and serve.

Nutrition:

Calories 274, Fat 12 g, Carbs 15.7 g, Protein 24.8 g

Zucchini Fritters

Preparation Time: 15 minutes

Cooking Time: 7 minutes

Serving: 4

Ingredients:

- 10-1/2 oz. zucchini, grated and squeezed
- 7 oz. Halloumi cheese
- 1/4 cup all-purpose flour
- Two eggs
- One teaspoon fresh dill, minced
- Salt and ground black pepper

Directions:

1. In a large bowl and mix together all the ingredients.
2. Make a small-sized patty from the mixture.
3. Press the Power Button of Air Fry Oven and turn the dial to select the Air Fry mode.

4. Press the Time button and again turn the dial to set the cooking time to 7 minutes.

5. Now push the Temp button and rotate the dial to set the temperature at 355 degrees F.

6. Press the Start/Pause button to start.

7. When the unit beeps to show that it is preheated, open the lid.

8. Arrange fritters into grease Sheet Pan and insert them in the oven.

9. Serve warm.

Nutrition:

Calories 253, Fat 17.2 g, Carbs 10 g, Protein 15.2 g

Air Fryer Hard-Boiled Eggs

Preparation Time: 1 minute

Cooking Time: 15 minutes

Serving: 6

Ingredients

- Six eggs

Directions:

1   Place the eggs in the air fryer basket. (You can put the eggs in an oven-safe bowl if you are worried about them rolling around and breaking.)

2   Set the temperature of your AF to 250°F. Set the timer and bake for 15 minutes (if you prefer a soft-boiled egg, reduce the cooking time to 10 minutes). Meanwhile, fill a medium mixing bowl half full of ice water. Use tongs to remove the eggs from the air fryer basket and transfer them to the ice water bath. Let the eggs sit for 5 minutes in the ice water.

3   Peel and eat on the spot or
refrigerate for up to 1 week.

Nutrition: Calories: 72; Fat: 5g; Saturated fat: 2g;
Carbohydrate: 0g; Fiber: 0g; Sugar: 0g; Protein: 6g;
Iron: 1mg; Sodium: 70mg

Easy Air Fryer Baked Eggs With Cheese

Preparation Time: 2 minutes

Cooking Time: 6 minutes

Serving: 2

Ingredients

- Two large eggs

- Two tablespoons half-and-half, divided

- Two teaspoons shredded Cheddar cheese, divided

- Salt

- Freshly ground black pepper

Directions:

1   Lightly coat the insides of 2 (8-ounce) ramekins with cooking spray. Break an egg into each ramekin.

2   Add one tablespoon of half-and-half and one teaspoon of cheese to each ramekin. Season with salt and pepper. Using a fork, stir the

egg mixture. Set the ramekins in the air fryer basket.

3   Set the temperature of your AF to 330°F. Set the timer and bake for 6 minutes.

4   Check the eggs to make sure they are cooked. If they are not done, cook for 1 minute more and check again.

Bacon-And-Eggs Avocado

Preparation Time: 5 minutes

Cooking Time: 17 minutes

Serving: 1

Ingredients

- One large egg

- One avocado, halved, peeled, and pitted

- Two slices of bacon

- Fresh parsley, for serving (optional)

- Sea salt flakes, for garnish (optional)

Directions:

1. Spray the air fryer basket with avocado oil —preheat the air fryer to 320°F. Fill a small bowl with cold water.

2. Soft-boil the egg: Place the egg in the air fryer basket. Cook for 6 minutes for a soft yolk or 7 minutes for a cooked yolk. Transfer the egg to the bowl of cold water and let sit for 2 minutes. Peel and set aside. Use a spoon to carve out extra space in the avocado halves' center until

the cavities are big enough to fit the soft-boiled egg.

3. Cut an avocado in half, put a soft-boiled egg inside, so it looks whole outside

4. Starting at one end of the avocado, wrap the bacon around the avocado to completely cover it. Use toothpicks to hold the bacon in place. Place the bacon-wrapped avocado in the air fryer basket and cook for 5 minutes. Flip the avocado over and cook for another 5 minutes, or until the bacon is cooked to your liking. Serve on a bed of fresh parsley, if desired, and sprinkle with salt flakes, if desired.

5. Best served fresh—store extras in an airtight container in the fridge for up to 4 days. Reheat in a preheated 320°F air fryer for 4 minutes, or until heated through.

Nutrition: Calories 536; Fat 46g; Protein 18g; Total carbs 18g; Fiber 14g

Double-Dipped Mini Cinnamon Biscuits

Preparation Time: 15 minutes

Cooking Time: 13 minutes

Serving: 8

Ingredients

BISCUITS

- 2 cups blanched almond flour

- ½ cup Swerve confectioners'-style sweetener or equivalent amount of liquid or powdered

    Sweetener

- One teaspoon baking powder

- ½ teaspoon acceptable sea salt

- ¼ cup plus two tablespoons (¾ stick) very cold unsalted butter

- ¼ cup unsweetened, unflavored almond milk

- One large egg

- One teaspoon vanilla extract

- Three teaspoons ground cinnamon

GLAZE:

- ½ cup Swerve confectioners'-style sweetener or equivalent amount of powdered sweetener

- ¼ cup heavy cream or unsweetened, unflavored almond milk

Directions:

1   Preheat the air fryer to 350°F. Line a pie pan that fits into your air fryer with parchment paper.

2   In a medium-sized bowl, mix the almond flour, sweetener (if powdered; do not add liquid sweetener), baking powder, and salt. Cut the butter into ½-inch squares, and then use a hand mixer to work the butter into the dry ingredients. When you are done, the mixture should still have chunks of butter.

3   In a small bowl, whisk together the almond milk, egg, and vanilla extract (if using

liquid sweetener, add it as well) until blended. Using a fork, stir the wet ingredients into the dry ingredients until large clumps form. Add the cinnamon and use your hands to swirl it into the dough. Form the dough into sixteen 1-inch balls and place them on the prepared pan, spacing them about ½ inches apart. (If you're using a smaller air fryer, work in batches if necessary.)

4   Bake in the air fryer until golden, 10 to 13 minutes. Remove from the air fryer and let cool on the pan for at least 5 minutes.

5   While the biscuits bake, make the glaze: Place the powdered sweetener in a small bowl and slowly stir in the heavy cream with a fork. When the biscuits have cooled somewhat, dip the tops into the glaze, allow it to dry a bit, and then dip again for thick ice. Serve warm or at room temperature.

6   An airtight container will preserve the cookies in the refrigerator for three

days. For more extended storage, pop cookies in the freezer for up to 3 months.

7   Preheat at 350°F air fryer for 5 minutes, or until warmed through, and dip in the glaze as instructed above.

Nutrition: Calories 546; Fat 51g; Protein 14g; Total carbs 13g; Fiber 6g

Foolproof Air Fryer Bacon

Preparation Time: 5 minutes

Cooking Time: 10 minutes

Serving: 5

Ingredients

- Ten slices bacon

Direction:

1   Cut the bacon slices in half so that they will fit in the air fryer.

2   Place the half-slices in the fryer basket in a single layer. (You may need to cook the bacon in more than one batch.)

3   Set the temperature of your AF to 400°F. Set the timer and fry for 5 minutes. Open the drawer and check the bacon. (The power of the fan may have caused the bacon to fly around during the cooking process. If so, use a fork or tongs to rearrange the slices.)

4   Reset the timer and fry for 5 minutes more. When the time has elapsed, recheck the bacon. If you like your bacon crispier, cook it for another 1 to 2 minutes.

Nutrition: Calories: 87; Fat: 7g; Saturated fat: 2g; Carbohydrate: 0g; Fiber: 0g; Sugar: 0g; Protein: 6g; Iron: 0mg; Sodium: 370mg

Merit Age Eggs

Preparation Time: 5 minutes

Cooking Time: 8 minutes

Serving: 2

Ingredients

- Two teaspoons unsalted butter (or coconut oil for dairy-free) for greasing the ramekins

- Four large eggs

- Two teaspoons chopped fresh thyme

- ½ teaspoon acceptable sea salt

- ¼ teaspoon ground black pepper

- Two tablespoons heavy cream (or unsweetened, unflavored almond milk for dairy-free)

- 3tablespoons finely grated Parmesan

- Fresh thyme leaves, for garnish (optional)

Directions:

1   Preheat the air fryer to 400°F.

Grease two 4-ounce ramekins with the butter. Crack two eggs into each ramekin and divide the thyme, salt, and pepper between the ramekins. Pour one tablespoon of the heavy cream into each ramekin. Sprinkle each ramekin with 1½ tablespoons of the Parmesan cheese.

2   Place the ramekins in the air fryer and cook for 8 minutes for soft-cooked yolks (longer if you desire a harder yolk). Garnish with a sprinkle of ground black pepper and thyme leaves, if desired. Best served fresh.

Nutrition: Calories 331; Fat 29g; Protein 16g; Total carbs 2g; Fiber 0.2g

Easy Air Fryer Buttermilk Biscuits

Preparation Time: 5 minutes

Cooking Time: 5 minutes

Serving: 12

Ingredients

- 2 cups all-purpose flour

- One tablespoon baking powder

- ¼ teaspoon baking soda

- 2teaspoons sugar

- One teaspoon salt

- 6tablespoons (¾ stick) cold unsalted butter, cut into 1-tablespoon slices

- ¾ cup buttermilk

- 4tablespoons (½ stick) unsalted butter, melted (optional)

Directions:

1. Spray the air fryer basket with olive oil.

2. In a large mixing bowl, combine the flour, baking powder, baking soda, sugar, and salt and mix well.

3. I am using a fork, cut in the butter until the mixture resembles a coarse meal.

4. Add the buttermilk and mix until smooth. Sprinkle flour on a clean work surface. Turn the dough out onto the work surface and roll it out until it is about ½ inch thick.

5. Using a 2-inch biscuit cutter, cut out the biscuits. Place the uncooked biscuits in the greased air fryer basket in a single layer.

6. Set the temperature of your AF to 360°F. Set the timer and bake for 5 minutes.

7. Transfer the cooked biscuits from the air fryer to a platter. Brush the tops with melted butter, if desired. Cut the remaining biscuits (you may have to gather up the dough scraps and reroll the dough for the last couple of biscuits). Bake the remaining biscuits.

8. Plate, serve, and enjoy!

Nutrition: (1 biscuit): Calories: 146; Fat: 6g; Saturated fat: 4g; Carbohydrate: 20g; Fiber: 1g; Sugar: 2g; Protein: 3g; Iron: 1mg; Sodium: 280mg

Breakfast Pizza

Preparation Time: 5 minutes

Cooking Time: 8 minutes

Serving: 1

Ingredients

- Two large eggs

- ¼ cup unsweetened, unflavored almond milk

- ¼ teaspoon acceptable sea salt

- ⅛ teaspoon ground black pepper

- ¼ cup diced onions

- ¼ cup shredded Parmesan cheese

- Six pepperoni slices

- ¼ teaspoon dried oregano leaves

- ¼ cup pizza sauce, warmed, for serving

Directions:

1   Preheat the air fryer to 350°F.
Grease a six by 3-inch cake pan.

2   In a small bowl, use a fork to
whisk together the eggs, almond milk, salt, and
pepper. Add the onions and stir to mix. Pour the
mixture into the greased pan—top with the cheese
(if using), pepperoni slices (if using), and oregano.
Cook for 8 minutes, until the eggs are cooked to
your liking.

3   Loosen the eggs from the pan's
sides with a spatula and place them on a serving
plate. Drizzle the pizza sauce on top. Best served
fresh.

Nutrition: Calories 357; Fat 25g; Protein 24g; Total
carbs 9g; Fiber 2g

Easy Bacon

Preparation Time: 2 minutes

Cooking Time: 6 minutes

Serving: 2

Ingredients

- Four slices thin-cut bacon or beef bacon

Directions:

1. Spray the air fryer basket with avocado oil —preheat the air fryer to 360°F.

2. Place the bacon in the air fryer basket in a single layer; spaced about ¼ inches apart, cook for 4 to 6 minutes (thicker bacon will take longer). Check the bacon after 4 minutes to make sure it is not overcooking.

3. Best served fresh—store extras in an airtight container in the fridge for up to 4 days. Reheat in a preheated 360°F air fryer for 2 minutes, or until heated through.

Nutrition: Calories 140; Fat 12g; Protein 8g; Total carbs 0g; Fiber 0g

Chicken And Asparagus

Preparation Time: 25 minutes

Cooking Time: 20 minutes

Serving: 4

Ingredients:

- 4chicken breasts, skinless; boneless and halved
- 1bunch asparagus; trimmed and halved
- 1 tbsp. Olive oil
- 1 tbsp. Sweet paprika
- Salt and black pepper to taste.

Directions:

1. Take a bowl and mix all the ingredients, toss, put them in your air fryer's basket and cook at 390°f for 20 minutes

2. Divide between plates and serve.

Nutrition:

Calories: 230; fat: 11g; fiber: 3g; carbs: 5g; protein: 12g

Spinach And Olives

Preparation Time: 25 minutes

Cooking Time: 20 minutes

Serving: 4

Ingredients:

- **½ cup tomato puree**
- 4cups spinach; torn
- **2cups black olives pitted and halved**
- **3celery stalks; chopped.**
- **1red bell pepper; chopped.**
- **Two tomatoes; chopped.**
- **Salt and black pepper**

Directions:

1. In a pan that fits your air fryer, mix all the ingredients except the spinach, toss, introduce the pan to the air fryer and cook

at 370°f for 15 minutes

2. Add the spinach, toss, cook for 5 - 6
   minutes more, divide into bowls and
   serve.

Nutrition:

Calories: 193; fat: 6g; fiber: 2g; carbs: 4g; protein: 6g

Broccoli Stew

Preparation Time: 20 minutes

Cooking Time: 15 minutes

Serving: 4

Ingredients:

- 1broccoli head, florets separated

- ¼ cup celery; chopped.

- ¾ cup tomato sauce

- 3spring onions; chopped.

- 3tbsp. Chicken stock

- Salt and black pepper

Directions:

1. In a pan that fits your air fryer, mix all the ingredients, toss, introduce the pan in your fryer and cook at 380°f for 15 minutes

2. Divide into bowls and serve for lunch.

Nutrition:

Calories: 183; fat: 4g; fiber: 2g; carbs: 4g; protein: 7g

Turkey And Bok Choy

Preparation Time: 25 minutes

Cooking Time: 20 minutes

Serving: 4

Ingredients:

- 1turkey breast, boneless, skinless, and cubed

- 2cups bok choy; torn and steamed

- 1tbsp. Balsamic vinegar

- 2tsp. Olive oil

- ½ tsp. Sweet paprika

- Salt and black pepper to taste.

Directions:

1. Take a bowl and mix the turkey with the oil, paprika, salt, and pepper, toss, transfer them to your air fryer's basket and cook at 350°f for 20 minutes

2. In a salad, mix the turkey with all the other ingredients, toss and serve.

Nutrition:

Calories: 250; fat: 13g; fiber: 3g; carbs: 6g; protein: 14g

Breakfast Potatoes

Preparation Time: 10 minutes

Cooking Time: 40 minutes

Serving: 2

Ingredients

- Potatoes 1 1/2 pounds

- Onion ¼ sliced

- Garlic cloves 2

- Green bell pepper 1

- Olive oil 1 Tablespoon

- Paprika 1/2 teaspoon

- Pepper 1/4 teaspoon

- Salt 1/2 teaspoon

Directions:

1. Clean the potatoes and bell pepper.

2. Dice the potatoes and boil them for 30 minutes in water. Pat dry after 30 minutes.

3. Chop the mushrooms, cabbage, and bell pepper. Garlic is minced.

4. In a bowl, put all the ingredients and combine them. Put it into an air-fryer.

5. Cook in an air fryer for 10 minutes at 390-400 degrees. Flip the bowl cook for another 5-10 minutes.

Breakfast Egg Rolls

Preparation Time: 10 minutes

Cooking Time: 25 minutes

Serving: 4

Ingredients

- Salt and pepper

- Milk 2 T

- Eggs 2

- Cheddar cheese ½ cup

- Olive oil one tablespoon

- Egg rolls 6

- Sausage patties 2

- Water

Directions:

1. Cook the sausage in a small skillet or replace it according to the packet. Remove and cut into bite-sized bits from the skillet.

2. Combine the chickens, sugar, and a touch of salt and pepper. Over medium / low flame, adds a teaspoon of oil or a little

butter to a plate. Pour in the egg mixture and fry, stirring regularly to render scrambled eggs for a few minutes. Stir the sausage in. Only put back.

3. Put the egg roll wrapper on a working surface to create a diamond formation with points. Position roughly 1 T of the cheese on the bottom third of the wrapper. Comb with a blend of chickens.

4. Water the finger or pastry brush and rub all the egg roll wrapper's sides, allowing it to close.

5. Fold the egg roll up and over the filling at the bottom stage, attempting to keep it as close as you can. Then, fold the sides together to make an envelope-looking form. Last, tie the whole wrapping around the top. Put the seam side down and begin the remaining rolls to assemble.

6. Heat the fryer for 5 minutes to 400 F.

7. Rub rolls with grease or spray them. Set the hot oven bowl in place. Set for 8

minutes to 400 F.

8. Flip over the egg rolls after 5 minutes. For a further 3 minutes, return the egg rolls to the air fryer.

Air Fryer Sausage Breakfast Casserole

Preparation Time: 10 minutes

Cooking Time: 45 minutes

Serving: 4

Ingredients

- Onion ¼ cup

- Red Bell pepper 1

- Green Bell pepper 1

- Breakfast sausage 1 lb.

- Hash Browns 1 lb.

- Eggs 4

- Yellow Bell pepper 1

Directions:

1. Foil fills the air fryer's basket.

2. Cover the uncooked sausage with it.

3. Put the peppers and onions uniformly on top.

4. Cook for 10 minutes at 355 *.

5. Open an air fryer and, if necessary, blend the casserole a little.

6. In a bowl, crack every egg, and then pour it right in the middle of the casserole.

7. Cook for another 10 minutes on 355 *.

8. To try, mix with salt and pepper.

Air Fryer Egg In Hole

Preparation Time: 10 minutes

Cooking Time: 15 minutes

Serving: 1

Ingredients

- Egg 1
  - Salt and pepper
  - Toast piece 1

Directions:

1. Spray the safe pan of the air fryer with nonstick oil spray.

2. Put a slice of bread in a healthy pan inside the air fryer.

3. Create a spot and then slice the bread with a cup.

4. Into the hole, crack the egg.

5. Fry for 6 minutes at 330 degrees, then use a large spoon and rotate the egg and fry for another 4 minutes.

Air Fryer Baked Egg Cups With Spinach & Cheese

Preparation Time: 10 minutes

Cooking Time: 30minutes

Serving: 4

Ingredients

- Milk 1 tablespoon

- Cheese 1-2 teaspoons

- Egg 1 large

- Frozen spinach one tablespoon

- Cooking spray

- Salt and black pepper

Directions:

1. Spray with oil spray inside the silicone muffin cups.

2. In a muffin cup, incorporate the cream, potato, spinach, and cheese.

3. Gently combine the egg whites with the liquids without separating the yolk and salt and pepper to taste.

4. For around 6-12 minutes, Air Fried at 330 ° F (single egg cups typically take about five minutes-several or doubled cups require as many as 12.

5. It may take a bit longer to cook in a ceramic ramekin. Cook for less time if you like runny yolks. After 5 minutes, regularly check the eggs to make sure the egg is of your desired texture.

Breakfast Casserole

Preparation Time: 10 minutes

Cooking Time: 55 minutes

Serving: 8

Ingredients:

- 1 lb. bacon, chopped
- One tablespoon olive oil
- Ten eggs
- ½ cup heavy cream
- 1 cup milk
- One teaspoon garlic powder
- One onion, diced
- 2 Roma tomatoes, seeded and chopped
- One green bell pepper, seeded and chopped
- 1 cup white cheddar, shredded
- ½ cup mozzarella cheese, shredded

- 28 oz. hash browns, frozen and shredded

- Salt and black pepper, to taste

Directions:

1. Grease a baking tray with cooking spray.

2. Heat oil in a skillet over medium heat. Add bacon and cook for 8 minutes. Add onion and cook for 3 minutes.

3. Whisk milk, eggs, cream, and garlic powder in a bowl—season with salt and pepper. Add onion, bell pepper, tomatoes, bacon, and cheddar cheese.

4. Add a layer of hash browns to the bottom of the tray. Add the egg mixture over the hash browns. Top with mozzarella.

5. Position the baking tray in Rack Position 2 and select the Bake setting. Set the temperature to 350 F and the time to 50 minutes. Serve.

Nutrition:

548 calories; 42 g fat; 18 g total carbs; 23 g protein

Cheesy Bacon And Egg Hash

Preparation Time: 10 minutes

Cooking Time: 35 minutes

Serving: 4

Ingredients:

- 7 oz. diced bacon, trimmed fat
- 24 oz. potatoes, scrubbed and peeled
- Two tablespoons olive oil
- Two scallions, trimmed and sliced
- ¼ cup Mozzarella cheese, shredded
- Four eggs
- Salt, pepper, to taste

Directions:

1. Cut potatoes into small cubes.

2. Arrange the potatoes in a single layer on a baking pan. Grease with cooking spray and position the baking pan in Rack

Position 2.

3. Select the Bake setting. Set the temperature to 30 and the time to 400F. Stir once halfway.

4. Remove from the oven, add bacon, and bake for 10 minutes.

5. Make four wells in the hash and add an egg into each well. Add mozzarella around each egg. Add the pan back to the oven and bake until eggs are done. Serve.

Nutrition:

413 calories; 28 g fat; 18 g total carbs; 17 g protein

Bacon Cheddar Biscuits

Preparation Time: 10 minutes

Cooking Time: 95 minutes

Serving: 8

Ingredients:

- One tablespoon baking powder
- Four slices of bacon
- 3 ½ cup all-purpose flour
- ½ teaspoon baking soda
- Two teaspoons granulated sugar
- ½ cup cheddar cheese, shredded
- One ¼ cup buttermilk, chilled
- ¼ cup green onions, sliced
- 1 cup + 2 tablespoons unsalted butter
- Two teaspoons kosher salt

Directions:

1. Add bacon to a baking pan. Position the baking pan in Rack Position 2 and select the Bake setting. Set the temperature to 375 F and the time to 20 minutes. Drain on paper towels and chop once cool.

2. Whisk baking powder, flour, baking soda, sugar, and salt in a bowl. Cut 1 cup cold butter into 1/8" pieces. Add few butter slices into flour and stir well to break the butter pieces. Freeze the mixture for 15 minutes.

3. Add cheddar cheese, bacon, and green onions to flour mixture. Stir well.

4. Add one ¼ cups buttermilk into the flour mixture and stir well. Knead the biscuit mixture a few times.

5. Dust a surface with flour and divide the dough into two parts.

6. Roll out the dough into a 1" thick square. Cut dough into four even-shaped squares and stack on top of each other. Leave ¼" border along the edges. Use a biscuit

cutter to form cookies.

7. Add to a baking pan and repeat with the remaining dough. Refrigerate for 30 minutes before baking.

8. Melt two tablespoons of butter and brush on top of each biscuit. Sprinkle with salt.

9. Position the baking pan in Rack Position 2 and select the Bake setting. Set the temperature to 450 F and the time to 15 minutes.

10.   Cool for 10 minutes. Serve.

Nutrition:

410 calories; 21.4 g fat; 44 g total carbs; 9 g protein

Potato Hash Brown Casserole

Preparation Time: 15 minutes

Cooking Time: 75 minutes

Serving: 12

Ingredients:

- 1 lb. sausages, casings removed
- One large sweet potato, peeled and diced into ½" chunks
- One red onion, chopped
- Two bell peppers, deseeded and diced
- One teaspoon garlic, minced
- 2 cups baby spinach leaves, washed
- 1 cup mushrooms, sliced
- 1 cup grape tomatoes, halved
- Ten eggs
- 1/3 cup milk
- 2/3 cup mozzarella cheese, shredded
- Salt and black pepper, to taste

Directions:

1. Grease a casserole dish with cooking spray.

2. Heat 1 tablespoon oil in a skillet over medium heat. Add sweet potatoes and fry for 2 minutes, stirring. Cover with lid and cook for 10 minutes, stirring occasionally. Transfer to the casserole dish.

3. Fry sausage meat in the skillet and break it up. Cook until done. Add garlic and onion and fry until onion is transparent. Add mushrooms and peppers and cook for 3 minutes, stirring occasionally.

4. Add spinach and cook until it wilts. Season well. Transfer veggies and sausages to the dish. Add sliced tomatoes and mix all ingredients.

5. Whisk eggs in a bowl with 1/3 cup cheese and milk.

6. Add the eggs over the casserole dish. Add remaining 1/3 cup cheese. Season well.

7. Position the oven to reach in Rack Position 1 and place the dish on top. Select the Bake setting. Set the temperature to 375 F and the time to 45 minutes.

8. Cool slightly. Slice and serve.

Nutrition:

248 calories; 15.2 g fat; 12 g total carbs; 18 g protein

Sweet Potato Casserole

Preparation Time: 10 minutes

Cooking Time: 35 minutes

Serving: 8

Ingredients:

- ½ cup granulated sugar

- 4 cups sweet potatoes, cooked and peeled

- ¼ cup unsalted butter

- ¼ cup milk

- Two teaspoons pure vanilla extract

- Two large eggs whisked

- ½ teaspoon salt

- ½ cup light brown sugar

- ½ cup all-purpose flour

- Two tablespoons unsalted butter

- ½ cup pecans, crushed

- Two tablespoons cinnamon sugar

- ½ teaspoon salt

Directions:

1. Grease a baking pan with cooking spray.

2. Mix sweet potatoes with milk, sugar, vanilla, ¼ cup butter, eggs, and ½ teaspoon salt in a bowl. Spread on a baking pan

3. Mix brown sugar, flour, butter, pecans, and salt in a separate bowl. Mix well. Add evenly over the sweet potatoes. Top with cinnamon sugar.

4. Position the baking pan in Rack Position 2 and select the Bake setting. Set the temperature to 350 F and the time to 25 minutes.

5. Select the Broil setting. Set the temperature to Broil and the time to 10. Serve.

Nutrition: 225 calories; 11 g fat; 34 g total carbs; 4 g protein

Cheesy Garlic Sweet Potatoes

Preparation Time: 10 minutes

Cooking Time: 45 minutes

Serving: 8

Ingredients:

- ¼ cup garlic butter, melted

- Four sweet potatoes halved lengthwise

- ¾ cup Mozzarella cheese, shredded

- ½ cup Parmesan cheese, grated

- Two tablespoons parsley, chopped

- Sea salt and black pepper, to taste

Directions:

1. Brush potatoes with garlic butter and season well with salt and pepper. Place cut side down on a greased baking pan.

2. Position the baking pan in Rack Position 2 and select the Bake setting. Set the temperature to 425 F and the time to 30 minutes.

3. Remove from the oven, flip and top with parsley, mozzarella and parmesan.

4. Select the Broil setting. Set the temperature to Broil and the time to 2 minutes. Season well and serve.

Nutrition:162 calories; 9 g fat; 13 g total carbs; 5 g protein

Blueberry Muffins

Preparation Time: 10 minutes

Cooking Time: 20 minutes

Serving: 12

Ingredients:

- One egg

    - 1 cup + 1 tablespoon all-purpose flour, unbleached

    - 1 ½ teaspoons baking powder

    - Four tablespoons unsalted butter

    - ¾ cup granulated sugar

    - ¼ cup whole milk

    - ½ teaspoon pure vanilla extract

    - 1 cup blueberries, fresh

    - ¼ teaspoon kosher salt

    - Pinch ground cinnamon

    - Cooking spray

Directions:

1. Add baking powder, 1 cup flour, salt, and cinnamon into a bowl. Whisk to combine well.

2. Mix sugar and butter until it becomes creamy.

3. Put the vanilla extract, and egg then mix it well.

4. Mix dry ingredients with wet ingredients. Stir well to combine. Mix blueberries with one tablespoon flour and add to the batter. Combine.

5. Grease a 6 cup muffin tray with cooking spray. Add the butter to the tin.

6. Position the oven to reach in Rack Position 1 and place the tin on top. Select the Bake setting. Set the temperature to 325 F and the time to 20 minutes. Serve.

Nutrition: 269 calories; 10 g fat; 17 g total carbs; 15 g protein

Eggs, Bacon, Tomato, And Cheese Bake

Preparation Time: 10 minutes

Cooking Time: 30 minutes

Serving: 8

Ingredients:

- ¼ cup extra-virgin olive oil

- 1 lb. bakery white bread, cut into 1" cubes

- One onion, halved and sliced

- 1 lb. sliced apple wood-smoked bacon, cut into ½" pieces

- 28 oz. Can whole Italian tomatoes, drained, chopped, and patted dry

- ½ lb. extra-sharp cheddar, shredded

- ½ teaspoon red pepper, crushed

- ½ lb. Monterey Jack cheese, shredded

- Two tablespoons snipped chives

- One ¾ cups chicken broth

- Eight eggs

- Salt, to taste

Directions:

1. Grease a baking dish with cooking spray. Toss bread with olive oil in a bowl and arrange on a baking pan.

2. Position the baking pan in Rack Position 2 and select the Bake setting. Set the temperature to 350 F and the time to 20 minutes, tossing twice.

3. Cook bacon in a skillet for 8 minutes over high heat. Drain the bacon and reserve two tablespoons fat in the skillet. Add onions to the skillet and cook for 5 minutes over medium heat. Add crushed red pepper and tomatoes and cook for 3 minutes.

4. Add the toasted bread cubes back to the bowl. Add the skillet contents along with shredded cheeses, bacon, broth, and chives. Stir okay—season with salt. Spread the mixture in the baking dish.

5. Position the oven to reach in Rack Position 1 and place the dish on top. Select the Bake setting. Set the temperature to 350 F and the time to 45 minutes.

6. Remove the baking dish from the oven and make eight wells in the bread mixture. Crack the egg into each well and return the container to the range—Bake for 15 minutes. Serve.

Nutrition: 953 calories; 57.9 g fat; 61 g total carbs; 47 g protein

Bacon Bombs

Preparation Time: 10 minutes

Cooking Time: 16 minutes

Serving: 4

Ingredients:

- Three center-cut bacon slices

- Three large eggs, lightly beaten

- 1 oz. 1/3-less-fat cream cheese softened

- 1 tbsp. chopped fresh chives

- 4 oz. fresh whole-wheat pizza dough

- Cooking spray

Directions:

1. Sear the bacon slices in a skillet until brown and crispy, then chop into fine crumbles. Add eggs to the same pan and cook for 1 minute, then stir in cream cheese, chives and bacon. Mix well, and then allow this egg filling to cool down.

2. Spread the pizza dough and slice into four -5inches circles. Divide the egg filling on top of each process and seal its edge to make dumplings.

3. Place the bacon bombs in the Air Fryer basket and spray them with cooking oil. Set the Air Fryer basket inside the Air Fryer toaster oven and close the lid.

4. Select the Air Fry mode at 350 degrees F temperature for 6 minutes. Serve warm.

Nutrition:

Calories: 278 Protein: 7.9gCarbs: 23gFat: 3.9g

Morning Potatoes

Preparation Time: 10 minutes

Cooking Time: 23 minutes

Serving: 4

Ingredients:

- Two russet potatoes, washed & diced

- ½ tsp. salt

- 1 tbsp. Olive oil

- ¼ tsp. garlic powder

- Chopped parsley, for garnish

Directions:

1. Soak the potatoes in cold water for 45 minutes, then drain and dry them—Toss potato cubes with garlic powder, salt, and olive oil in the Air Fryer basket.

2. Set the Air Fryer basket inside the Air Fryer toaster oven and close the lid. Select the Air Fry mode at400 degrees F

temperature for 23 minutes.

3. Toss them well when cooked halfway through, and then continue cooking.

4. Garnish with chopped parsley to serve.

Nutrition:

Calories: 146   Protein: 6.2gCarbs: 41.2gFat: 5g

Breakfast Pockets

Preparation Time: 10 minutes

Cooking Time: 10minutes

Serving: 6

Ingredients:

- One box puff pastry sheet
- Five eggs
- ½ cup loose sausage, cooked
- ½ cup bacon, cooked
- ½ cup cheddar cheese, shredded

Directions:

1. Stir cook egg in a skillet for 1 minute and then mix with sausages, cheddar cheese, and bacon. Spread the pastry sheet and cut it into four rectangles of equal size.

2. Divide the egg mixture over each rectangle. Fold the edges around the filling and seal them. Place the pockets in the Air Fryer basket.

3. Set the Air Fryer basket inside the Air Fryer toaster oven and close the lid.

4. Select the Air Fry mode at 370 degrees F temperature for 10 minutes. Serve warm

Nutrition:

Calories: 387   Protein: 14.6gCarbs: 37.4gFat: 6g

Avocado Flautas

Preparation Time: 10 minutes

Cooking Time: 24 minutes

Serving: 8

Ingredients:

- 1 tbsp. butter
- Eight eggs, beaten
- ½ tsp. Salt
- ¼ tsp. pepper
- 1 ½ tsp. cumin
- 1 tsp. chili powder
- Eight fajita-size tortillas
- 4 oz. cream cheese softened
- Eight slices of cooked bacon
- Avocado Crème:
- Two small avocados
- ½ cup sour cream
- One lime, juiced

- ½ tsp. Salt

- ¼ tsp. pepper

Directions:

1. In a skillet, melt butter and stir in eggs, salt, cumin, pepper, and chili powder, then stir cook for 4 minutes. Spread all the tortillas and top them with cream cheese and bacon. Then divide the egg scramble on top and finally add cheese.

2. Roll the tortillas to seal the filling inside. Place four rolls in the Air Fryer basket. Set the Air Fryer basket inside the Air Fryer toaster oven and close the lid. Select the Air Fry mode at 400 degrees F temperature for 12 minutes.

3. Cook the remaining tortilla rolls in the same manner. Meanwhile, blend avocado crème ingredients in a blender, then serve with warm flautas.

Nutrition:

Calories: 212   Protein: 17.3gCarbs: 14.6gFat: 11.8g

Cheese Sandwiches

Preparation Time: 10 minutes

Cooking Time: 10 minutes

Serving: 2

Ingredients:

- One egg

- 3 tbsp. Half and half cream

- ¼ tsp. vanilla extract

- Two slices sourdough, white or multigrain bread

- 2½ oz. sliced Swiss cheese

- 2 oz. sliced deli ham

- 2 oz. cut deli turkey

- 1 tsp. butter, melted

- Powdered sugar

- Raspberry jam, for serving

Directions:

1. Beat egg with half and half cream and vanilla extract in a bowl. Place one bread slice on the working surface and top it

with ham and turkey slice and Swiss cheese.

2. Place the other bread slice on top, then dip the sandwich in the egg mixture, then place it in a suitable baking tray lined with butter. Set the baking tray inside the Air Fryer toaster oven and close the lid.

3. Select the Air Fry mode at 350 degrees F temperature for 10 minutes. Flip the sandwich and continue cooking for 8 minutes. Slice and serve.

Nutrition:

Calories: 412   Protein: 18.9gCarbs: 43.8gFat: 24.8g

Sausage Cheese Wraps

Preparation Time: 10 minutes

Cooking Time: 10 minutes

Serving: 4

Ingredients:

- Eight sausages

- Two pieces American cheese, shredded

- 8-count refrigerated crescent roll dough

Directions:

1. Roll out each crescent roll and top it with cheese and one sausage. Fold both the crescent sheet's top and bottom edges to cover the link and roll it around the sausage.

2. Place four rolls in the Air Fryer basket and spray them with cooking oil. Set the Air Fryer basket inside the Air Fryer toaster oven and close the lid. Select the Air Fry mode at 380 degrees F temperature for 3 minutes.

3. Cook the remaining rolls in the same manner. Serve fresh.

Nutrition:

Calories: 296   Protein: 34.2gCarbs: 17gFat: 22.1g

Chicken Omelet

Preparation Time: 10 minutes

Cooking Time: 18 minutes

Serving: 4

Ingredients:

- Four eggs
- ½ cup chicken breast, cooked and diced
- 2 tbsp. Shredded cheese, divided
- ½ tsp. Salt divided
- ¼ tsp. Pepper divided
- ¼ tsp. Granulated garlic, divided
- ¼ tsp. onion powder, divided

Directions:

1. Spray two ramekins with cooking oil and keep them aside. Crack two large eggs into each ramekin, and then add cheese and seasoning.

2. Whisk well, and then add ¼ cup chicken. Place the ramekins in a baking tray.

3. Set the baking tray inside the Air Fryer toaster oven and close the lid. Select the Bake mode at 330 degrees F temperature for 18 minutes. Serve warm.

Nutrition:

Calories: 322   Protein: 17.3gCarbs: 4.6gFat: 21.8g

Sausage Burritos

Preparation Time: 10 minutes

Cooking Time: 10 minutes

Serving: 6

Ingredients:

- Six medium flour tortillas
- Six scrambled eggs
- ½ lb. ground sausage, browned
- ½ bell pepper, minced
- 1/3 cup bacon bits
- ½ cup shredded cheese
- Oil, for spraying

Directions:

1. Mix eggs with cheese, bell pepper, bacon, and sausage in a bowl. Spread each tortilla on the working surface and top it with ½ cup egg filling.

2. Roll the tortilla like a burrito, then place three burritos in the Air Fryer basket.

103

3. Spray them with cooking oil. Set the Air Fryer basket inside the Air Fryer toaster oven and close the lid. Select the Air Fry mode at 330 degrees F temperature for 5 minutes.

4. Cook the remaining burritos in the same manner. Serve fresh.

Nutrition:

Calories: 197   Protein: 7.9gCarbs: 58.5gFat: 15.4g

Sausage Patties

Preparation Time: 10 minutes

Cooking Time: 20 minutes

Serving: 4

Ingredients:

- 1.5 lbs. ground sausage
- 1 tsp. chili flakes
- 1 tsp. dried thyme
- 1 tsp. Onion powder
- ½ tsp. each paprika and cayenne
- Sea salt and black pepper, to taste
- 2 tsp. brown sugar
- 3 tsp. minced garlic
- 2 tsp. Tabasco
- Herbs for garnish

Directions:

1. Toss sausage ground with all the spices, herbs, sugar, garlic, and Tabasco sauce in a bowl. Make 1.5-inch-thick and 3-inch round patties out of this mixture.

2. Place the sausage patties in the Air Fryer basket. Set the Air Fryer basket inside the Air Fryer toaster oven and close the lid. Select the Air Fry mode at 370 degrees F temperature for 20 minutes.

3. Flip the patties when cooked halfway through, and then continue cooking.

Nutrition:

Calories: 208   Protein: 24.3gCarbs: 9.5gFat: 10.7g

Spicy Sweet Potato Hash

Preparation Time: 10 minutes

Cooking Time: 16 minutes

Serving: 4

Ingredients

- Two large sweet potatoes, diced

- Two slices bacon, cooked and diced

- 2 tbsp. olive oil

- 1 tbsp. smoked paprika

- 1 tsp. of sea salt

- 1 tsp. ground black pepper

- 1 tsp. dried dill weed

Directions

1. Toss sweet potato with all the spices and olive oil in the Air Fry basket. Set the Air Fryer basket inside the Air Fryer toaster oven and close the lid.

2. Select the Air Fry mode at 400 degrees F temperature for 16 minutes. Toss the potatoes after every 5 minutes.

3. Once done, toss in bacon and serve warm.

Nutrition:

Calories: 134   Protein: 6.6gCarbs: 36.5gFat: 6g

Lightning Source UK Ltd.
Milton Keynes UK
UKHW050020200822
407522UK00015B/123